Zero Waste Revolution

"Your Roadmap to Living Eco-Friendly"

By, Bishwajit Saha

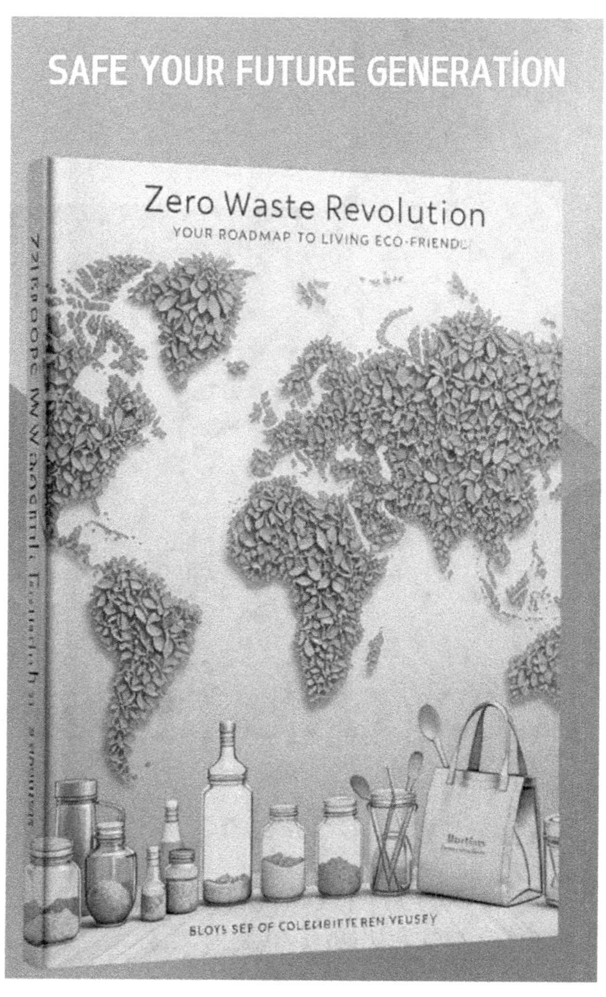

Published By: Mrs. Shilpi Saha

ISBN:

Content

Introduction:

Why Zero Waste Living Matters

In an age of growing awareness about climate change and environmental degradation, the zero-waste lifestyle has emerged as a powerful way to take action. It is not just a trend but a transformative approach to living that prioritizes sustainability, mindfulness, and responsibility. This book, **"Zero Waste Revolution: Your Roadmap to Living Eco-Friendly,"** is your guide to embarking on a journey that can improve your life and help the planet thrive.

The Big Picture: Understanding the Environmental Crisis

The modern world generates waste at an alarming rate. According to studies, over **2 billion tons of solid waste** are produced annually worldwide, and much of this waste ends up in landfills or pollutes our oceans. The plastic we discard today can take **hundreds of years to decompose**, often breaking down into microplastics that harm marine life and infiltrate our food systems.

The consequences of this waste crisis are profound:

1. **Environmental Degradation**: Overflowing landfills emit methane, a potent greenhouse gas, contributing significantly to global warming.

2. **Health Impacts**:

   Chemicals from improperly disposed of waste contaminate soil and water, leading to health problems in communities worldwide.

3. **Resource Depletion**:

   The linear model of "take, make, dispose" depletes natural resources at unsustainable rates.

Reflective Prompt: Take a moment to think about your daily habits. How much waste do you generate? Write down three areas where you notice waste in your life (e.g., plastic packaging, food waste, or fast fashion).

Inspirational Quote:

"We do not inherit the Earth from our ancestors; we borrow it from our children." - *Native American Proverb*

Benefits of Zero Waste Living

Living a zero-waste lifestyle is about more than just reducing trash. It's about reimagining how we interact with the world around us. Here are some of the key benefits:

1. **Saving Money**:

   - Buying reusable products means spending less on disposable items over time.

   - Reducing food waste and cooking at home can significantly lower grocery bills.

   - Second-hand shopping and upcycling save money while giving items a new life.

2. Health Benefits:

- o Opting for natural, non-toxic products reduces exposure to harmful chemicals found in plastics and cleaning agents.

- o Eating fresh, unpackaged foods encourages a healthier diet.

3. Environmental Impact:

- o Cutting down on waste reduces pollution and conserves resources like water and energy.

- o Supporting sustainable practices helps protect ecosystems and biodiversity.

Real-Life Example:

Meet Sarah, a mother of two who transformed her family's lifestyle by embracing zero waste. By switching to cloth diapers, composting kitchen scraps, and buying in bulk, Sarah reduced her household waste by 80% and saved over $1,200 in one year.

Inspirational Quote:

"The greatest threat to our planet is the belief that someone else will save it." - Robert Swan

What This Book Will Help You Achieve

This book is your comprehensive roadmap to living an eco-friendly life. It's designed to make the transition to zero waste manageable and inspiring. Whether you're new to sustainability or looking to deepen your commitment, this guide will help you:

1. **Understand the Zero Waste Movement**: Learn the principles and philosophies that underpin this lifestyle.

2. **Identify and Reduce Waste**: Discover practical ways to cut down on waste in every area of your life, from your kitchen to your wardrobe.

3. **Adopt Sustainable Habits**: Develop habits that align with your values and contribute to long-term change.

4. **Save Money While Saving the Planet**: Find ways to live sustainably without breaking the bank.

5. **Inspire Others**: Share your journey and inspire friends, family, and your community to join the revolution.

Daily Exercise:

Start a journal to track your zero-waste journey. Write down one small change you can make today to reduce waste—perhaps bringing a reusable bag to the store or swapping a disposable water bottle for a reusable one. Reflect on how it makes you feel.

Closing Thought for the Introduction

The journey to zero waste is not about perfection but progress. It's about taking small, meaningful steps that collectively lead to significant change. As you turn the pages of this book, you'll discover that living sustainably is not only achievable but immensely rewarding. Together, we can redefine what it means to live well, leaving a legacy of hope and resilience for future generations.

Inspirational Quote:

"Small acts, when multiplied by millions of people, can transform the world." - Howard Zinn

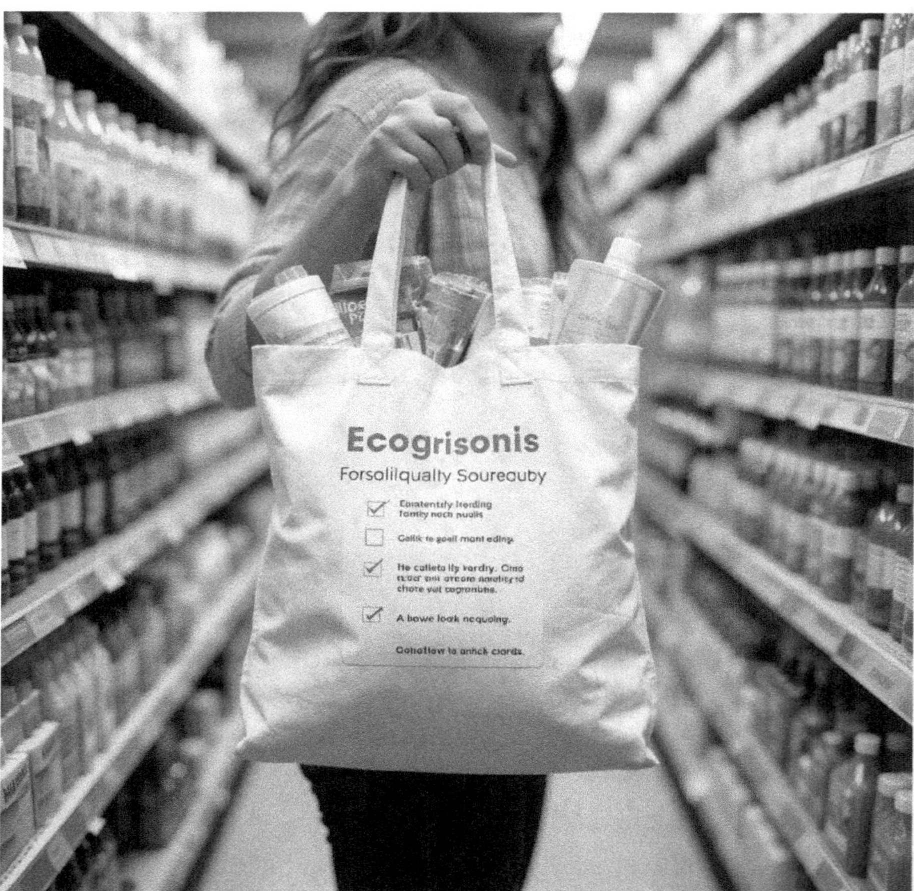

Chapter 1

Assess Your Current Waste Habits

The first step toward a zero-waste lifestyle is understanding your current habits and their impact on the environment. By assessing your waste footprint, identifying problem areas, and setting realistic goals, you create a solid foundation for meaningful change. This chapter will guide you through practical steps to evaluate and reshape your relationship with waste.

What Is Your Waste Footprint? Conducting a Waste Audit

To embark on your zero-waste journey, you must first understand how much waste you generate and where it comes from. A waste audit is a simple but powerful tool that provides insight into your consumption patterns.

How to Conduct a Waste Audit

1. **Gather Supplies**: Prepare gloves, a notebook, and separate bins or bags for categorizing waste.

2. **Track Your Waste**: Over a week, collect and categorize everything you discard. Common categories include:

- o **Food waste** (e.g., leftovers, peels, expired food)

- o **Plastics** (e.g., packaging, bottles, wrappers)

- o **Paper** (e.g., mail, receipts, napkins)

- o **Textiles** (e.g., old clothes, fabrics)

- o **Miscellaneous** (e.g., electronics, household items)

3. **Analyse the Data**: At the end of the week, review your waste. Identify patterns, such as frequent use of single-use items or excessive food waste.

Detailed Steps

- **Daily Observation**: Make note of items you discard regularly. Is it packaging from snacks, or uneaten leftovers?

- **Weigh Your Waste**: If possible, weigh your daily waste to understand its volume. This helps in quantifying your impact.

- **Involve Your Household**: Encourage family or roommates to participate, as their habits contribute to the overall waste.

Reflective Prompt

Take 15 minutes to review your waste audit results. Ask yourself:

- What surprised you most about the waste you generated?

- Which category was the largest contributor?

- How did conducting the audit make you feel?

Inspirational Quote

"You cannot change what you are unaware of, but once you are aware, you cannot ignore it." –

Identifying Problem Areas

After conducting a waste audit, it's time to pinpoint specific areas where waste accumulates. These are your "problem areas," and addressing them is critical for success.

Common Problem Areas

1. Food Waste:

- o **The Scale of the Problem**: Globally, up to **30% of food is wasted**, contributing significantly to landfill waste and greenhouse gas emissions.

- o **Practical Solutions**: Implement meal planning, buy only what you need, and learn to preserve food through freezing or pickling.

- o **Tools**: Use apps like "Too Good to Go" or "OLIO" to save surplus food.

2. Single-Use Plastics:

- o **Examples**: Straws, grocery bags, coffee cups, and packaging account for significant environmental harm.

- o **Practical Solutions**: Invest in reusable alternatives such as stainless-steel straws, cloth shopping bags, and glass jars. Shop at bulk stores when possible.

3. Fast Fashion:

- o **Impact**: The fashion industry contributes to **10% of global carbon emissions** and produces waste that takes decades to decompose.

- o **Practical Solutions**: opt for second-hand stores, repair and upcycle clothing, or participate in clothing swaps.

4. Household Waste:

- o **Examples**: Disposable cleaning products, paper towels, excessive packaging from online orders.

- o **Practical Solutions**: Replace with reusable cloths, biodegradable alternatives, and buy in bulk to minimize packaging.

Real-Life Example

James, a college student, discovered during his waste audit that he used over 30 plastic bottles a month. By switching to a reusable water bottle and refilling it from campus fountains, he saved money and significantly reduced his waste footprint.

Reflective Prompt

Think about your daily routine. Which of the problem areas resonate most with your lifestyle? Write down three changes you could make to reduce waste in those areas.

Inspirational Quote

"Do the best you can until you know better. Then when you know better, do better." – Maya Angelou

Setting Realistic Goals

Change doesn't happen overnight. Setting achievable goals tailored to your lifestyle ensures long-term success and prevents overwhelm.

How to Set Realistic Goals

1. **Start Small:**

   - Focus on one problem area at a time. For example, replace disposable coffee cups with a reusable mug before tackling other changes.

2. **Make SMART Goals:**

   - **Specific:** "I will eliminate single-use plastic bags from my shopping routine."

   - **Measurable:** "I will track my usage over the next 30 days."

   - **Achievable:** "I will buy reusable bags and keep them in my car."

   - **Relevant:** "Reducing plastic aligns with my goal to live sustainably."

- o **Time-bound**: "I will achieve this goal by the end of the month."

3. **Celebrate Milestones**:

   - o Recognize progress, no matter how small. This keeps you motivated.

Detailed Examples

- **Example 1**: Laura, a working professional, started by composting her kitchen scraps. Over six months, she expanded her efforts to eliminate single-use plastics and shop locally.

- **Example 2**: Miguel aimed to stop using disposable coffee cups. By the end of three months, he had inspired his coworkers to do the same by gifting them reusable mugs.

Daily Exercise

Write down three specific goals you'd like to achieve in the next month. For each goal, outline the steps you'll take and how you'll measure success.

Inspirational Quote

"A journey of a thousand miles begins with a single step." – Lao Tzu

Closing Thought for Chapter 1

Understanding your waste habits is the cornerstone of a zero-waste lifestyle. By conducting a waste audit, identifying problem areas, and setting realistic goals, you're not only taking control of your environmental impact but also paving the way for a more mindful and sustainable life. Remember, every small change adds up to a big difference.

Inspirational Quote:

"The Earth is what we all have in common." – Wendell Berry

Chapter 2: The 5 Rs of Zero Waste Living

At the heart of zero-waste living is a framework known as the 5 Rs: Refuse, Reduce, Reuse, Recycle, and Rot. Each "R" represents a practical and actionable step toward minimizing waste and living an eco-friendlier life. This chapter dives deeply into each principle, offering insights, exercises, and real-world examples to help you integrate these habits into your daily life.

Refuse: Saying No to Things You Don't Need

Refusing is the first and most impactful step. By saying no to unnecessary items, you prevent waste from entering your life in the first place.

How to Practice Refusal

1. **Decline Single-Use Items:**

   o   Say no to plastic straws, disposable cutlery, and paper napkins. Carry reusable alternatives instead.

2. **Avoid Freebies:**

   o   Free samples, promotional items, and unnecessary gifts often become clutter and waste.

3. **Opt Out of Junk Mail:**

- o Register with services that reduce unsolicited mail and switch to digital statements.

Daily Exercise

Track how many items you refuse in a week. Note the situations and think about the alternatives you used or could have used.

Reflective Prompt

Reflect on a time you said no to an unnecessary item. How did it feel, and what impact do you think it made?

Inspirational Quote

"The greatest wealth is to live content with little." – Plato

Reduce: Simplifying and Minimizing Consumption

Reducing involves cutting down on what you consume and using resources more efficiently.

Practical Steps to Reduce

1. **Buy Less, Choose Well**:
   - o Invest in high-quality items that last longer rather than buying cheap, disposable products.

2. **Embrace Minimalism**:
   - o Declutter your home and focus on items that add value to your life.

3. **Reduce Packaging Waste**:
   - o Shop at bulk stores, use refill stations, and choose products with minimal packaging.

Real-Life Example

Sarah, a teacher, started buying second-hand furniture and repairing old appliances instead of replacing them. Over a year, she saved $1,200 and significantly reduced her waste.

Reflective Prompt

Identify one area in your life where you could reduce consumption. What steps can you take this week to make a change?

Inspirational Quote

"Do what you can, with what you have, where you are." – Theodore Roosevelt

Reuse: Opting for Reusable Items Over Disposables

Reusing is about making the most of what you already have and choosing durable, reusable options instead of disposables.

Ways to Reuse

1. **Switch to Reusables:**
   - Use stainless steel water bottles, cloth grocery bags, and glass food containers.

2. **Repurpose Old Items:**
   - Turn old clothes into cleaning rags or glass jars into storage containers.

3. **Shop Second-Hand:**
   - Visit thrift stores and online marketplaces for pre-loved items.

Real-Life Example

John, a college student, started using a reusable coffee cup and was inspired to create a campus initiative promoting reusable containers.

Daily Exercise

Choose three disposable items in your daily routine and find reusable alternatives. Note how this change impacts your life.

Inspirational Quote

"Reuse it or lose it." – Unknown

Recycle: The Do's and Don'ts of Effective Recycling

Recycling is an essential step but often misunderstood. Doing it correctly ensures that materials can be processed and reused.

The Basics of Recycling

1. **Know Your Local Rules:**

   o Learn what can and cannot be recycled in your area.

2. **Clean and Sort:**

   o Rinse items to avoid contamination and sort them appropriately.

3. **Avoid Wish-Cycling:**

   o Don't toss non-recyclable items into the recycling bin, hoping they'll be recycled.

Real-Life Example

Emma, a mother of two, educated her family on proper recycling. They reduced their landfill waste by 30% within six months.

Reflective Prompt

Review your current recycling habits. Are there any mistakes you've been making? How can you improve?

Inspirational Quote

"Recycling is a good start, but reducing and reusing are better." – Unknown

Rot: Starting a Composting Habit for Organic Waste

Composting, or "rotting," is the process of turning organic waste into nutrient-rich soil. It's a natural way to dispose of food scraps and yard waste.

How to Start Composting

1. **Choose a Method:**

   o   Options include backyard composting, worm bins, or municipal composting programs.

2. **Know What to Compost:**

   o   Include fruit and vegetable scraps, coffee grounds, and yard waste. Avoid meat, dairy, and oily foods.

3. **Maintain Your Compost:**

   o   Balance green (wet) and brown (dry) materials, and aerate the pile regularly.

Real-Life Example

Carlos, an apartment dweller, started a worm composting bin under his sink. He reduced his food waste by 50% and used the compost for his balcony garden.

Daily Exercise

Start collecting your organic waste for composting. Research composting options that fit your living situation.

Inspirational Quote

"Composting is the ultimate recycling." – Unknown

Closing Thought for Chapter 2

The 5 Rs of zero-waste living provide a clear and actionable roadmap for reducing waste and living sustainably. By refusing unnecessary items, reducing consumption, reusing durable alternatives, recycling effectively, and composting organic waste, you're taking significant steps toward a healthier planet and a more mindful lifestyle.

Inspirational Quote:

"What we do today, right now, will have an accumulated effect on all of our tomorrows." – Alexandra Stoddard

Chapter 3
Simplify Your Home

Your home is more than a physical space; it is a sanctuary, a reflection of your lifestyle, and a cornerstone of your well-being. Simplifying your home isn't just about cleaning and organizing—it's about creating a space that aligns with your values and promotes sustainability. This chapter will guide you through the transformative journey of decluttering, organizing, and cultivating a minimalist mindset, equipping you with the tools to design an intentional and eco-friendly living space.

Declutter with Purpose: Sustainable Methods of Decluttering

Decluttering is often viewed as a one-time task, but with a purpose-driven approach, it becomes a lifestyle choice that aligns with zero-waste living. The goal isn't just to tidy up but to do so mindfully and sustainably, ensuring items are responsibly reused, repurposed, or recycled.

Understanding the Why Behind Clutter

Before diving into decluttering, reflect on why clutter exists in your home. Is it a result of impulsive purchases, emotional attachments, or a lack of organization systems? By identifying the root cause, you can create lasting change.

Eco-Friendly Decluttering Strategies

1. **The "Joyful" Test**:
   Inspired by Marie Kondo's philosophy, hold each item and ask yourself if it sparks joy. For a zero-waste twist, consider whether it also serves a practical purpose or aligns with your sustainable values.

2. **Plan Donation Drops Strategically**:
   Avoid sending items to landfills by donating them to local charities, shelters, or online swap groups. For clothing, organizations like *Goodwill* or *Dress for Success* ensure items are reused meaningfully.

3. **Upcycle Unusable Items**:

   o   Old jars become plant holders.

   o   Torn clothes can be repurposed as cleaning cloths.

   o   Worn-out books can transform into creative home decor.

4. **Set Realistic Goals**:
   Dedicate 15–30 minutes daily to decluttering one area. Focus on steady progress instead of attempting to overhaul your home in one go.

Daily Exercise

Pick a drawer, shelf, or corner and spend 20 minutes decluttering. Reflect on how your choices impact the environment and your mindset.

Real-Life Example

Meera, a mother of two, found her kitchen overflowing with unused gadgets. By applying these techniques, she donated her extra appliances to a local cooking school, recycled broken items responsibly, and upcycled glass jars for spice storage. The result was a clutter-free, functional kitchen that felt welcoming.

Reflective Prompt

Think about an item you've been holding onto. What emotional or practical value does it have? How could letting it go create space for something more meaningful?

Inspirational Quote

"Clutter isn't just physical stuff. It's old ideas, toxic relationships, and

bad habits. Clutter is anything that doesn't support your better self." – Eleanor Brownn

Zero Waste Organizing Tips: Using Baskets, Jars, and Second-Hand Finds

Once you've decluttered, the next step is creating an organization system that is both functional and sustainable. Zero-waste organizing isn't about buying more containers; it's about using resources creatively and mindfully.

Principles of Sustainable Organization

1. **Reuse Before Buying**:
   - Glass jars from pasta sauces or pickles can store pantry staples.
   - Baskets from old gift hampers make excellent storage solutions.

2. **Seek Multipurpose Items**:
   - Vintage wooden crates can double as bookshelves or toy storage.
   - Second-hand furniture can be repurposed to suit new needs, like turning an old ladder into a towel rack.

3. **Think Beyond Plastic**:
   - opt for materials like wood, glass, and metal that are durable and eco-friendly.

4. **Label with Care**:

  o Reusable labels made from chalkboard stickers or upcycled paper ensure your systems remain adaptable.

Organization Tips for Key Spaces

- **Kitchen**: Use stackable jars for grains and cereals. Store utensils in ceramic mugs or old tins.

- **Closet**: Implement the "one in, one out" rule—when you buy something new, donate or repurpose an older item.

- **Living Room**: Keep it simple with baskets for blankets and books. Avoid over-decorating to maintain a minimalist aesthetic.

Real-Life Example

Sophie, an artist, transformed her cluttered studio by repurposing wine crates into paint and canvas storage. She used glass jars to organize her brushes and upcycled an old dresser as a standing easel. This eco-friendly approach enhanced her creative flow while reducing waste.

Reflective Prompt

What items in your home are underutilized? How can you repurpose them to bring order and utility to your space?

Inspirational Quote

"Have nothing in your house that you do not know to be useful or believe to be beautiful." – William Morris

Creating a Minimalist Mindset: Focus on Quality Over Quantity

Minimalism is more than a design choice—it's a philosophy that emphasizes intentional living. By valuing quality over quantity, you not only simplify your home but also reduce waste and make environmentally conscious decisions.

The Mindset Shift

1. **Redefine "Enough"**:

   - Challenge the consumer culture of more-is-better. Instead, ask yourself, "What do I truly need to live comfortably and sustainably?"

2. **Quality Over Quantity**:

   - Invest in fewer, high-quality items that last longer, such as durable cookware, versatile clothing, and well-crafted furniture.

3. **Detach from Trends**:

   - Avoid the pressure of keeping up with fleeting trends. Focus on timeless designs and materials that age gracefully.

Benefits of Minimalism

- **Financial Freedom**: Buying less frees up money for experiences and investments.

- **Environmental Impact**: Fewer purchases mean fewer resources used and less waste generated.

- **Mental Clarity**: A minimalist home creates a peaceful environment that reduces stress and enhances focus.

Real-Life Example

Rahul, a tech enthusiast, transitioned to a minimalist lifestyle by selling outdated gadgets and limiting new purchases to essential, high-quality tools. This shift reduced his electronic waste and improved his financial stability.

Daily Exercise

Identify three items in your home that represent quantity over quality. Consider whether you could replace them with a more durable or functional alternative in the future.

Reflective Prompt

Write about a time you chose quality over quantity. How did it make you feel, and how can you apply this mindset to other areas of your life?

Inspirational Quote

"Simplicity is the ultimate sophistication." – Leonardo da Vinci

Bringing It All Together

Simplifying your home is an ongoing journey that requires mindfulness and intention. By decluttering purposefully, organizing sustainably, and embracing minimalism, you create a living space that reflects your values and supports a zero-waste lifestyle.

Action Steps Recap

1. Declutter one space at a time and dispose of items responsibly.

2. Repurpose what you have and invest in sustainable organizing solutions.

3. Shift your mindset to value quality over quantity.

Closing Reflection

Imagine your home as a sanctuary—a place that nurtures your well-being while treading lightly on the planet. Each small change you make contributes to a larger movement toward sustainability and simplicity.

Inspirational Quote

"Out of clutter, find simplicity. From discord, find harmony. In the middle of difficulty lies opportunity." – Albert Einstein

Chapter 4

Waste-Free Grocery Shopping

Planning Ahead: Creating Sustainable Shopping Lists

Planning your shopping is the cornerstone of zero-waste living. It saves time, reduces waste, and ensures you're intentional with your purchases.

The High Cost of Impulse Buys

A 2023 study found that 20% of grocery budgets are spent on unplanned purchases. Many of these items end up in the trash. With a sustainable shopping list, you can avoid this trap and feel good about every item in your cart.

Enhanced Tips for Planning

1. **Use Technology to Your Advantage:**
   Apps like Paprika, Mealtime, and Yummly help you plan meals, generate shopping lists, and even suggest recipes based on what's already in your pantry.

2. **Batch Prep with a Purpose:**
   Consider meals that can be prepped in advance, like soups or stir-fries, to reduce waste from spoiled ingredients.

3. **Involve the Family:**
   Turn planning into a family activity. Let kids help choose recipes or take responsibility for checking pantry items. This builds awareness from an early age.

Daily Reflection Prompt

Take a moment to consider how much food you throw away each week. What could you change about your planning to waste less?

Choosing the Right Stores: Farmers' Markets, Bulk Bins, and Local Co-ops

Shopping at the right places can transform the way you shop. These stores offer fresher, less-packaged options while supporting sustainable practices.

The Farmers' Market Experience

Picture a bustling farmers' market: the sun shining on piles of vibrant tomatoes, the earthy smell of fresh herbs, and the friendly chatter of local farmers sharing recipes. Shopping here isn't just an errand—it's an experience.

Tips for Maximizing Farmers' Market Trips

- **Bring Your Own Containers**: Some vendors allow you to use jars or cloth bags for purchases like berries or grains.

- **Arrive Early or Late**: Early birds get the best selection, but latecomers often find discounts on unsold produce.

Navigating Bulk Bins

Bulk bins can be intimidating at first. What if you don't know how much to scoop? How do you weigh items? Most stores have staff who are happy to help—don't hesitate to ask.

Pro Tip: Write the item code on your jar with a washable marker to streamline checkout.

Co-Ops for Community Support

In 2024, co-ops have seen a resurgence as communities prioritize local, sustainable economies. Joining one often comes with perks like discounts and member-exclusive products.

Ditching Plastic: Reusable Bags, Produce Sacks, and Alternatives

Plastic is convenient but devastating to the planet. Thankfully, there are countless ways to avoid it during grocery shopping.

Beyond Bags

Reusable bags are just the beginning. Consider alternatives for all types of packaging:

- **Mesh Produce Bags**: Lightweight and washable.

- **Silicone Food Bags**: Great for buying and storing small items.

- **Glass or Stainless-Steel Containers**: Ideal for deli purchases.

DIY Solutions for Budget-Conscious Shoppers

Can't afford new reusable items? Repurpose old pillowcases into produce bags or wash and reuse glass jars from store-bought items.

Addressing Plastic-Free Challenges

Switching to a plastic-free lifestyle takes effort. Not every store offers bulk options, and some items are nearly impossible to find without packaging. Focus on progress, not perfection. Replace one habit at a time, and celebrate every win.

Inspirational Quotes and Final Thoughts

- *"We don't need a handful of people doing zero waste perfectly. We need millions of people doing it imperfectly."* — Anne-Marie Bonneau

By adopting waste-free grocery shopping, you contribute to a brighter, cleaner future. Small steps lead to big changes, and your choices inspire those around you.

Call to Action

Commit to one change from this chapter today. Whether it's planning your meals, visiting a farmers' market, or ditching plastic, every effort matters. Together, we can create a revolution.

Chapter 5

Cooking and Eating the Zero Waste Way

Cooking is a daily activity that can either contribute to waste or act as a catalyst for sustainable living. This chapter explores how you can transform your kitchen habits, reduce waste, and cultivate a meaningful connection with the food you consume.

Meal Planning: Preventing Food Waste with Smarter Prep

The Foundation of Zero Waste Cooking

Planning is the cornerstone of a zero-waste kitchen. Without a clear plan, it's easy to buy excess food, let produce spoil, or fall into the trap of takeout meals that come with disposable packaging.

Detailed Strategies for Smarter Meal Prep

1. **Analyse Your Habits**
   Take note of what you usually buy and what ends up wasted. Are you purchasing too many perishable items? Do you overestimate how much you'll cook during the week? Adjust your shopping habits based on this analysis.

2. **The Art of Flexible Recipes**
   Create meal plans that accommodate changes. For instance, plan a vegetable stir-fry that can use any mix of veggies you have on hand. Flexibility reduces the likelihood of ingredients going to waste.

3. **Portion Control**
   Prepare meals in portions that match your household's eating habits. Over-preparation often leads to leftovers that aren't consumed in time.

4. **Prep Like a Pro**
   Spend one day a week prepping ingredients: wash and chop vegetables, portion out snacks, and pre-cook staples like grains and beans. This reduces midweek stress and ensures you use what you've purchased.

Daily Exercise

Write down a meal plan for the week that incorporates at least three items already in your pantry or fridge. Reflect on how this changes your shopping habits and reduces waste.

Creative Leftovers: Repurposing Scraps and Avoiding Waste

Rethinking "Scraps"

The term "scraps" often implies useless leftovers, but in a zero-waste kitchen, scraps are opportunities. With a little creativity, these byproducts can enhance meals and reduce waste.

Innovative Ways to Use Scraps

1. **Stocks and Broths**
   Collect veggie peels, onion skins, and herb stems in a freezer bag. Once you have enough, simmer them with water for a homemade stock.

2. **Bread Revival**
   Stale bread can become croutons, breadcrumbs, or even bread pudding.

3. **Fruit Preservation**
    Overripe bananas are perfect for smoothies or baking, while soft apples can be turned into applesauce or pie filling.

4. **Herb Longevity**
    Blend wilting herbs with olive oil and freeze in ice cube trays for ready-to-use flavour boosters.

Enhanced Real-Life Example

Lila, an eco-conscious chef, turned her food scraps into a thriving part of her menu. She uses vegetable trimmings for soups, potato peels for crisps, and citrus rinds for infused oils. Her approach has saved her hundreds of dollars annually and inspired her customers to adopt similar habits.

New Reflective Prompt

What scraps do you often throw away? Can they be repurposed, stored, or donated instead?

Composting Kitchen Waste: A Beginner's Guide to Composting

The Role of Composting in a Sustainable Kitchen

Even with impeccable planning and creative cooking, some food waste is inevitable. Composting is the natural next step, ensuring that nothing goes to waste.

Expanded Composting Methods

1. **Traditional Backyard Composting**
    A simple compost bin or heap in your backyard can handle most kitchen waste. Layer food scraps with yard waste to maintain balance and aerate regularly to speed up decomposition.

2. **Vermicomposting**
    Worm bins are excellent for small spaces. Red wigglers digest organic matter, creating rich compost called castings, perfect for gardening.

3. **Bokashi Composting**
   This anaerobic method ferments food scraps, including meat and dairy, into pre-compost that can be buried in soil to complete decomposition.

4. **Electric Composters**
   If you're short on time or space, electric composters like Lomi or Vitamix Food Cycler quickly break down waste into soil-like material with minimal effort.

Expanded Troubleshooting Tips

- **Odor Issues**:
  Use a compost activator or add shredded newspaper to absorb excess moisture.

- **Slow Decomposition**:
  Chop larger scraps into smaller pieces to speed up the process.

- **Pest Control**:
  Add a secure lid or bury food scraps deep within the compost pile.

Inspirational Add-On

"Composting turns waste into wealth by giving back to the Earth. Each peel, rind, or core contributes to a cycle of renewal."

Connecting Food Choices to the Bigger Picture

Zero-waste cooking is about more than preventing waste—it's a mindset shift. It encourages respect for the resources that go into producing food, from the farmer's labour to the water and soil used to grow it.

Expanded Call to Action

This week, try one new habit: start a compost bin, repurpose a leftover, or plan meals more intentionally. Share your journey with others to inspire a ripple effect.

Final Touches for Engagement

Daily Zero-Waste Challenge

Create a zero-waste dinner using only items already in your kitchen. Bonus points if you incorporate food scraps!

Quote for Reflection

"The journey to sustainability begins at the dinner table."

Chapter 6

Zero Waste Bathroom and Personal Care

Introduction

The bathroom is a hotspot for single-use plastics, synthetic chemicals, and unnecessary waste. This chapter aims to transform your bathroom into a zero-waste haven, emphasizing eco-friendly products, DIY solutions, and sustainable choices. By adopting these practices, you not only reduce your environmental impact but also improve your health and save money.

Section: Plastic-Free Products

Why Go Plastic-Free in the Bathroom?

Plastic waste from bathroom products often ends up in landfills or waterways. Toothbrushes, disposable razors, and single-use bottles contribute to the mounting environmental crisis. By switching to plastic-free alternatives, you align your personal care routine with a sustainable lifestyle.

List of Plastic-Free Essentials

1. **Bamboo Toothbrushes**
   Transitioning to a bamboo toothbrush is a simple yet impactful change. Choose brands that offer compostable bristles or send-back programs for recycling.

2. **Bar Soaps and Solid Toiletries**
   Beyond just shampoo and conditioner, explore solid toothpaste tablets, lotion bars, and shaving bars. These products are often sold without packaging or wrapped in compostable materials.

3. **Safety Razors**
   opt for stainless-steel safety razors that last for decades. These razors not only reduce plastic waste but also save you money in the long run.

4. **Plastic-Free Oral Care**

   o **Mouthwash Tablets**: Dissolvable tablets that eliminate the need for plastic bottles.

   o **Dental Floss**: Look for silk or bamboo floss in refillable glass containers.

5. **Eco-Friendly Toilet Paper**
   Consider toilet paper made from bamboo or recycled paper, packaged in plastic-free wrapping.

Additional Practical Tip

Use glass or stainless-steel dispensers for liquid soaps or oils. Refill them at bulk stores or online vendors that offer refill pouches.

DIY Personal Care

Why DIY?

Homemade personal care products are free from harmful chemicals, customizable to your preferences, and significantly reduce packaging waste. They also offer a sense of empowerment and creativity.

Recipes:

1. **DIY Toothpaste**

   o **Ingredients**: 2 tbsp baking soda, 1 tbsp coconut oil, 10 drops of peppermint essential oil.

   o **Method**: Mix the ingredients until smooth and store in a small glass jar.

2. **DIY Dry Shampoo**

   o **Ingredients**: Cornstarch, cocoa powder (for darker hair), and a few drops of essential oil.

   o **Method**: Blend and store in a shaker jar. Apply with a makeup brush for easy distribution.

3. **DIY Face Masks**

   o **Oatmeal Mask**: Blend oats with honey and a splash of water for a hydrating mask.

   o **Clay Mask**: Combine bentonite clay with apple cider vinegar for deep cleansing.

4. **DIY Body Scrub**

   o **Ingredients**: Used coffee grounds, sugar, and coconut oil.

   o **Method**: Mix and use as a natural exfoliant.

Practical Advice for Beginners

Start with one DIY product and refine the recipe based on your preferences. For instance, experiment with essential oils to create a scent profile you love.

Section: Sustainable Menstrual Products

The Case for Reusable Menstrual Products

Disposable menstrual products are not only wasteful but also expensive over time. Switching to reusables can save hundreds of dollars annually and drastically reduce your environmental footprint.

Detailed Overview of Options

1. **Menstrual Cups**

   o **Materials**: Made from medical-grade silicone or rubber, these cups are safe and long-lasting.

- o **Usage Tips**: Fold and insert like a tampon. Sterilize between cycles for hygiene.

2. **Reusable Pads**

   - o **Design**: Available in various sizes and absorbencies, reusable pads are made from organic cotton or bamboo.

   - o **Maintenance**: Rinse in cold water before machine washing.

3. **Period Underwear**

   - o **Brands**: Explore trusted brands offering different styles and absorbencies.

   - o **Care Instructions**: Wash in cold water and air dry for longevity.

Addressing Misconceptions

- **Myth**: Reusable products are messy.
  Reality: Modern designs ensure they're leak-proof and hygienic.

- **Myth**: They're expensive.
  Reality: While the initial investment may seem high, reusables pay for themselves in a few cycles.

Troubleshooting Tips and Real-Life Examples

Common Challenges and Solutions

1. **Challenge**: Struggling to transition to a menstrual cup.

   - o **Solution**: Start with a smaller size and practice during lighter flow days.

2. **Challenge**: DIY products not working as expected.

   - o **Solution**: Adjust ingredient proportions or try a different recipe.

Real-Life Success Stories

Meet Sophia, who reduced her bathroom waste by 80% in a year. She started with small changes, like a bamboo toothbrush, and gradually adopted reusable menstrual products and DIY skincare. Today, her bathroom is a plastic-free sanctuary.

Inspirational Quote

"Sustainability starts at home. Transform your bathroom into a space that nurtures both you and the planet."

Expanded Call to Action

This week, make one change in your bathroom. Whether it's switching to a bamboo toothbrush, trying a DIY recipe, or investing in reusable menstrual products, every step matters. Share your journey online to inspire others.

Chapter 7
Wardrobe Makeover – Sustainable Fashion

Fashion is more than just a means of self-expression—it's also a reflection of our values. Unfortunately, the fast fashion industry has become synonymous with environmental degradation, unethical labor practices, and overconsumption. In this chapter, we'll explore how to transform your wardrobe into a sustainable, stylish collection that supports both people and the planet.

The Problem with Fast Fashion: An In-Depth Look

Fast fashion's impact is staggering, and updated statistics underscore the urgency of change:

- **Environmental Impact:**
  - Produces 92 million tons of waste annually, equivalent to a garbage truck's worth dumped every second.
  - Textile dyeing is responsible for 20% of global wastewater pollution.
  - Polyester production emits three times more carbon dioxide than cotton.

- **Ethical Concerns**:
  - Over 170 million children are involved in child labour globally, many in garment production.
  - Recent exposés have revealed garment workers earning less than $1 per hour in hazardous conditions.

Global Diversity in Fast Fashion

Fast fashion's effects differ across regions. For instance:

- In the U.S., high consumption rates drive overproduction.
- In developing countries like Bangladesh, unsafe working conditions dominate discussions.

Building a Capsule Wardrobe: A Comprehensive Guide

The Capsule Wardrobe Concept

Seasonal Capsules: Break down wardrobe essentials by season to adapt to varying climates.

  - **Summer**: Linen tops, lightweight skirts, sandals.
  - **Winter**: Wool sweaters, thermal leggings, sturdy boots.

Leveraging Digital Tools

Modern apps make capsule wardrobe planning easier:

- **Stylebook**: Helps catalog your wardrobe and plan outfits.
- **Closet+**: Tracks usage to identify underused items.

Cultural Adaptations

Highlight culturally relevant capsule wardrobe staples:

- In India, saris and kurtas can be paired with versatile blouses and pants.
- In Japan, incorporating timeless kimonos with modern clothing creates a sustainable fusion.

Thrift, Repair, and Swap: Modern Solutions

Thrifting for a Digital Age

Online platforms have revolutionized second-hand shopping:

- **ThredUp** and **Poshmark**: Allow users to buy and sell pre-loved clothing globally.

- **Depop**: A hub for vintage and trendy finds.

Advanced Repair Techniques

Beyond simple sewing, explore innovative solutions:

- **Iron-On Patches**: Revive torn jeans with creative designs.

- **Fabric Glue**: A quick fix for seams and hems.

- **Repair Cafés**: Community events where volunteers fix clothes and teach repair skills.

Organizing Clothing Swaps

Detailed steps to host a successful event:

1. **Set Guidelines**: Ensure items are clean and in good condition.

2. **Create Themes**: Focus on specific styles or seasons to attract more participants.

3. **Use social media**: Promote the event through local groups or apps like Meetup.

Daily Practices for Sustainable Fashion

More Practical Tips

- **Wash Smarter**: Use a Guppy friend washing bag to catch microplastics from synthetic fabrics.

- **Choose Non-Toxic Detergents**: opt for biodegradable, eco-friendly detergents.

- **Care for Shoes and Accessories**: Polish leather shoes and repair broken zippers to extend their life.

A Month-Long Challenge

- **Week 1**: Inventory your wardrobe.

- **Week 2**: Thrift or swap for missing pieces.

- **Week 3**: Learn a new repair skill.

- **Week 4**: Plan a capsule wardrobe for the next season.

Refined Real-Life Success Stories

- **Case Study: Swap Meets in Singapore**
  Residents in Singapore host regular swap events in public spaces, reducing clothing waste by 30% in participating communities.

- **From Designer to Recycler**
  A French designer created a thriving business repurposing discarded clothing into high-end fashion, showcasing the potential for upcycling.

New Inspirational Quote

"Wear your values. When you choose sustainability, you choose a future where fashion is kind to people and the planet."

Improved Engagement with Reflective Prompts

1. **Reflect on Fast Fashion's Impact:**

   - How many items in your wardrobe are from fast fashion brands?

   - What changes can you make to reduce your dependency on them?

2. **Visualize Your Ideal Wardrobe**:

   o   What does your dream capsule wardrobe look like?

   o   List three pieces you could invest in to start building it.

3. **Repair and Repurpose Brainstorm**:

   o   What's the oldest piece in your wardrobe, and how can you make it new again?

Daily Practices for a Sustainable Wardrobe

1. **Pause Before Purchasing**

   o   Ask yourself: Do I really need this? Can I borrow or rent it instead?

2. **Care for Your Clothes**

   o   Wash with cold water, air dry when possible, and store items properly to extend their lifespan.

3. **Track Your Fashion Footprint**

   o   Use apps or tools to measure the environmental impact of your clothing choices.

Inspirational Quote

"Fashion should be about self-expression, not self-destruction. Choose timeless over trendy, sustainable over fleeting."

Call to Action

This week, take one step toward a sustainable wardrobe. Whether it's creating your capsule wardrobe, exploring a local thrift store, or repairing a favourite piece of clothing, every action counts. Share your progress with others and inspire them to join the zero-waste fashion revolution.

Chapter 8

Zero Waste Cleaning and Household Supplies

Cleaning and maintaining a household don't have to come at the expense of the planet. With simple changes and creative solutions, you can transition to a zero-waste approach that's kinder to the environment and your wallet. This chapter dives into DIY cleaning products, eco-friendly tools, and energy and water efficiency tips that empower you to live a greener life without sacrificing cleanliness or convenience.

DIY Cleaning Products: Recipes for Every Need

Switching to homemade cleaning products is one of the easiest ways to reduce household waste. Commercial cleaners often come in single-use plastic bottles and contain harsh chemicals that harm the environment. With a few simple ingredients, you can create effective, safe, and eco-friendly alternatives.

All-Purpose Cleaner

Ingredients:

- 1-part white vinegar

- 1 part water

- Lemon peel (optional)
- A few drops of essential oil (e.g., tea tree, lavender)

Instructions:

1. Combine all ingredients in a spray bottle.
2. Shake well before use.
3. Use on countertops, glass, and other surfaces (avoid marble or granite as vinegar may damage these).

Laundry Soap

Ingredients:

- 1 bar of castile soap (grated)
- 1 cup washing soda
- 1 cup baking soda
- 10–15 drops of essential oil (optional)

Instructions:

1. Mix all ingredients in a container.
2. Use 1–2 tablespoons per load.
3. Store in an airtight jar to maintain freshness.

Glass Cleaner

Ingredients:

- 1 cup rubbing alcohol
- 1 cup water
- 1 tablespoon white vinegar

Instructions:

1. Mix all ingredients in a spray bottle.
2. Spray onto glass surfaces and wipe with a microfiber cloth.

Natural Air Freshener

Ingredients:

- Water

- Essential oils (citrus, eucalyptus, or peppermint work well)

- A small spray bottle

Instructions:

1. Fill the bottle with water and add a few drops of essential oil.

2. Shake and spray around the home for a refreshing scent.

Eco-Friendly Tools: Sustainable Cleaning Alternatives

Switching to eco-friendly cleaning tools reduces waste and eliminates the need for disposable supplies.

Wooden Brushes

Why they're better:

- Biodegradable handles reduce landfill waste.

- Durable and versatile for scrubbing pots, pans, and floors.

Pro Tip: Choose brushes with replaceable bristles to extend their life.

Compostable Sponges

Replace synthetic sponges with options made from natural materials like loofah or cellulose.

- Compost them when worn out to complete the zero-waste cycle.

Cloth Rags Over Paper Towels

Reusable cloth rags made from old T-shirts or towels are excellent for cleaning spills and wiping surfaces.

- Wash and reuse instead of constantly buying paper towels.

Dusting Without Plastic

- Use wool or bamboo dusters that attract particles naturally.

- Washable duster heads reduce long-term costs.

Storage Tips for DIY Tools

- Organize cleaning supplies in glass jars or reusable containers.

- Label jars for easy identification and an aesthetically pleasing cleaning station.

Energy and Water Efficiency: Tips for Reducing Utility Waste

Cleaning sustainably goes beyond tools and products. Incorporating energy and water efficiency into your routine reduces both waste and utility bills.

Conserve Energy During Cleaning

- **Air Dry Clothes**: Use a drying rack or clothesline instead of a dryer.

- **Efficient Vacuuming**: Opt for vacuums with HEPA filters for cleaner air and energy savings.

Minimize Water Waste

- **Turn Off Taps**: Avoid leaving water running while scrubbing dishes or cleaning surfaces.

- **Fix Leaks**: A dripping faucet can waste up to 3,000 gallons of water a year.

- **Bucket Method for Floors**: Use a bucket of water for mopping instead of running water continuously.

Eco-Friendly Appliances

- **Energy-Efficient Washing Machines**: Choose machines with a high Energy Star rating.

- **Cold Water Washing**: Save energy by washing clothes in cold water.

Real-Life Example: The Zero-Waste Cleaning Challenge

A family of four in Portland committed to a zero-waste cleaning routine for one year. By switching to homemade products and reusable tools, they:

- Reduced household waste by 80%.

- Saved over $300 on cleaning supplies annually.

- Inspired their neighbours to adopt similar practices, creating a community-wide impact.

Their favourite tip? Hosting a DIY cleaning product workshop where neighbours shared recipes and techniques.

Daily Practices for Sustainable Cleaning

1. **Morning Ritual**: Start the day with a quick wipe-down using reusable cloths and your DIY all-purpose cleaner.

2. **Weekly Task**: Dedicate one day a week to refill your homemade cleaners and assess your tools.

3. **Monthly Check-In**: Track how much waste you've avoided and celebrate your progress.

Inspirational Quote

"A clean home and a clean planet go hand in hand. Every sustainable choice you make is a step toward a brighter, healthier future."

Reflective Prompts

1. **Audit Your Cleaning Supplies**:

   - How many single-use plastic items are in your cleaning stash?

   - Which items can you replace with sustainable alternatives this month?

2. **DIY Confidence Check**:

- o Which homemade cleaning product recipe are you most excited to try?

- o What challenges might you face, and how can you overcome them?

3. **Set a Goal**:

- o Choose one area of your cleaning routine to make completely zero-waste in the next 30 days.

Conclusion

Transitioning to zero-waste cleaning isn't just about reducing waste—it's about embracing a healthier, more cost-effective way of living. With simple DIY recipes, sustainable tools, and efficient practices, you can turn every cleaning task into a win for the environment. This chapter equips you with the knowledge and inspiration to make your household a shining example of eco-friendly living.

Let's clean green—because a sustainable future starts at home.

Chapter 9

Mindful Consumption: Buying Less and Buying Better

In a world overflowing with products and promises, adopting mindful consumption is a revolutionary act of sustainability. By understanding how to discern genuine eco-friendly claims, participating in challenges that reduce unnecessary spending, and prioritizing durable, high-quality items, you can transform your shopping habits into a powerful force for good. This chapter explores how to embrace a more intentional, thoughtful approach to consumption that benefits both the planet and your wallet.

Understanding Greenwashing: Spotting Fake Eco-Friendly Claims

In the quest for sustainable living, it's easy to fall for products that appear eco-friendly but are far from it. Greenwashing, a deceptive marketing practice, misleads consumers into believing a product or company is environmentally responsible when it isn't.

What Is Greenwashing?

Greenwashing occurs when brands use vague language, imagery, or claims to exaggerate their environmental benefits. Examples include:

- Using terms like "natural" or "eco-friendly" without clear evidence.

- Highlighting one green feature while ignoring other harmful aspects.

- Presenting certifications that aren't credible or are self-created.

How to Spot Greenwashing

- **Look for Transparency**: Legitimate companies provide detailed information about their sustainability efforts, including material sources, production processes, and third-party certifications.

- **Investigate Certifications**: Recognized eco-labels include Fair Trade, USDA Organic, and B Corporation.

- **Scrutinize Language**: Beware of vague claims like "green," "clean," or "earth-friendly." Genuine efforts are backed by data and specifics.

- **Research the Brand**: Check reviews, customer feedback, and independent assessments. Brands with a true commitment to sustainability are often celebrated by trusted organizations.

By learning to identify greenwashing, you can direct your spending power toward businesses genuinely working to protect the planet.

The Buy Nothing Challenge: A Guide to Buying Less for a Month

What if you stopped shopping for an entire month? The Buy Nothing Challenge is a powerful exercise in mindful consumption, helping you reassess your relationship with material goods and uncover new ways to meet your needs without buying new items.

Why Try the Challenge?

- **Reduce Waste**: Avoid impulse buys that end up in landfills.

- **Save Money**: A month of no spending can reveal how much you can save by curbing unnecessary purchases.

- **Foster Creativity**: Discover creative solutions to your needs, such as borrowing, swapping, or repurposing.

How to Start

1. **Set Clear Rules**: Define what counts as a "buy." Groceries and essential items like medicine are typically exempt.

2. **Prepare Mentally**: Expect moments of temptation and have strategies ready to resist, like revisiting your goals or reaching out to supportive friends.

3. **Track Your Progress**: Keep a journal of what you wanted to buy but didn't and how you solved the need without a purchase.

4. **Celebrate Success**: At the end of the month, reflect on how your habits and mindset have shifted.

What You'll Learn

Participants often report that the challenge is surprisingly liberating. It fosters a deeper appreciation for the items you already own and highlights the joy of connecting with others through sharing, borrowing, and gifting.

Investing in Quality: How Durable Products Save Money Over Time

The phrase "buy less, buy better" encapsulates the essence of sustainable consumption. By prioritizing quality over quantity, you not only reduce waste but also save money in the long run.

The True Cost of Cheap Products

Inexpensive, low-quality items may seem like a bargain, but they often:

- Wear out quickly, requiring frequent replacements.

- Create more waste, as discarded items pile up in landfills.

- Encourage overconsumption by providing a temporary, unsatisfying solution.

Benefits of Durable, High-Quality Products

- **Longevity**: Items made with care and robust materials last longer, reducing the need for replacements.

- **Cost Savings**: While the upfront cost may be higher, the long-term savings outweigh the initial expense.

- **Sustainability**: Fewer purchases mean fewer resources used and less waste generated.

How to Identify Quality Products

1. **Material Matters**: Choose natural, durable materials like stainless steel, wood, or organic cotton.

2. **Check Reviews**: Look for feedback from others about the product's durability and performance.

3. **Consider Warranties**: Companies confident in their products often offer warranties or repair services.

4. **Buy Timeless Designs**: Classic, versatile styles are less likely to go out of fashion or become obsolete.

Real-Life Story: A Mindful Consumer's Journey

Maria, a mother of three, decided to embrace mindful consumption after noticing how often her family threw away broken or unused items. She started by participating in the Buy Nothing Challenge, during which she borrowed tools from neighbours, swapped clothes with friends, and repurposed old furniture. Inspired by the challenge, Maria began investing in high-quality products, such as stainless-steel kitchenware and durable children's clothing.

After one year, Maria reduced her household waste by 60% and saved over $1,500. Her journey shows that buying less and buying better isn't just an eco-friendly choice—it's a financially and emotionally rewarding one too.

Daily Practices for Mindful Consumption

1. **Pause Before Purchasing**: Ask yourself if you truly need the item or if there's another way to fulfil the need.

2. **Opt for Second hand**: Check thrift stores or online marketplaces before buying new.

3. **Support Ethical Brands**: Choose companies committed to sustainability, fair labor practices, and transparency.

4. **Embrace Minimalism**: Focus on owning fewer, higher-quality items that bring real value to your life.

Reflective Prompts

1. **Audit Your Spending**:

   - What are your most frequent purchases?

   - How many of them are necessities versus wants?

2. **Set Intentional Goals**:

   - What one area of your life could you simplify by buying less?

   - What would you invest in if you committed to quality over quantity?

3. **Track Progress**:

   - Keep a record of items you avoided buying and the alternatives you used.

Inspirational Quote

"The most sustainable product is the one you never buy. But when you must, make it a choice that lasts a lifetime."

Conclusion

Mindful consumption isn't about deprivation—it's about making intentional, impactful choices. By learning to spot greenwashing, challenging yourself to buy nothing for a month, and committing to high-quality investments, you'll reduce waste, save money, and cultivate a lifestyle that aligns with your values. This chapter equips you with actionable strategies to shop smarter and live more sustainably, proving that less truly is more.

Let's redefine consumption together—because every mindful purchase moves us closer to a greener future.

Chapter 10
Community and Sharing Economy

Transitioning to a zero-waste lifestyle isn't just about individual efforts—it's about creating a collective impact. The sharing economy exemplifies the power of community in driving sustainability. By sharing instead of owning, hosting or participating in swap events, and using platforms that promote collaborative consumption, we can reduce waste, save money, and foster stronger connections. This chapter explores how to embrace these practices to build a greener, more connected world.

Sharing Instead of Owning: Libraries, Tool Swaps, and Community Gardens

The idea of sharing instead of owning is a cornerstone of sustainable living. Rather than accumulating items that are used infrequently, why not borrow, share, or access communal resources?

Libraries: Beyond Books

Libraries aren't just for avid readers anymore. Many now offer:

- **Tool Libraries**: Borrow drills, hammers, or gardening tools for occasional DIY projects.

- **Toy Libraries**: Access toys for children, reducing the need to buy and discard plastic playthings.

- **Kitchen Libraries**: Share high-cost or rarely used items like pasta makers, blenders, or specialty bakeware.

  Libraries reduce the demand for new products and provide access to quality items for everyone, fostering a sense of shared responsibility.

Tool Swaps

A tool swap allows people to exchange items they own but rarely use. Instead of buying an expensive tool for a one-time project, you can borrow or trade with someone in your community. Tool swaps can also include:

- Lawn equipment

- Camping gear

- Specialty tools like tile cutters or paint sprayers

Community Gardens

Community gardens transform urban spaces into lush, productive areas where neighbours grow food together. Benefits include:

- Reducing food miles by growing fresh, local produce.

- Strengthening community ties through shared labour and rewards.

- Teaching sustainable gardening practices to participants of all ages.

Hosting or Joining Swap Events: Clothes, Books, and Household Items

Swap events are a fun, engaging way to reduce waste while building connections. Whether you're exchanging clothes, books, or household items, swaps are a sustainable alternative to traditional shopping.

Why Swaps Work

- **Cost-Effective**: Participants save money by trading instead of buying.

- **Reduces Waste**: Extends the life of items, keeping them out of landfills.

- **Social Engagement**: Encourages interaction and collaboration among neighbours and friends.

How to Host a Swap Event

1. **Choose a Venue**: A community centre, park, or someone's home works well.

2. **Set the Theme**: Decide if the swap will focus on clothing, books, toys, or a mix of items.

3. **Establish Guidelines**: Create rules for item quality, maximum contributions, and how unclaimed items will be handled.

4. **Promote the Event**: Use social media, flyers, and word of mouth to invite participants.

5. **Create a System**: Arrange items neatly and set up tables or areas for specific categories to make browsing easier.

Swaps can be one-time events or regular gatherings, making them a cornerstone of a sharing-focused lifestyle.

Collaborative Consumption: Apps and Platforms That Encourage Sharing

Technology has revolutionized the sharing economy, making it easier than ever to participate in collaborative consumption. Apps and platforms connect people who need items or services with those willing to share or rent.

Popular Sharing Platforms

- **Peer-to-Peer Rentals**: Platforms like Fat Llama let you rent anything from cameras to kayaks.

- **Car Sharing**: Apps like Turo and Zipcar allow users to rent cars for short trips or specific needs.

- **Accommodation Sharing**: Airbnb and Couchsurfing provide alternatives to hotels, emphasizing shared spaces.

- **Ride Sharing**: Apps like Uber Pool and BlaBlaCar promote carpooling to reduce fuel consumption and costs.

Benefits of Collaborative Consumption

- **Eco-Friendly**: Reduces the need for mass production and resource extraction.

- **Economic Savings**: Sharing costs less than owning.

- **Convenience**: Access items or services only when needed, eliminating storage concerns.

How to Get Started

1. Explore platforms that align with your needs.

2. Begin by offering items or services you're willing to share.

3. Stay informed about local sharing opportunities and apps.

Real-Life Story: A Sharing Economy Success

Jack, a graphic designer, embraced the sharing economy after realizing he used many of his possessions only a few times a year. He joined a local tool library, participated in neighbourhood swap events, and listed his DSLR camera on a peer-to-peer rental app.

Not only did Jack save money by borrowing what he needed, but he also earned extra income from renting out his equipment. Through these experiences, he built meaningful relationships with his community, proving that sharing is not just sustainable—it's enriching.

Daily Practices for Embracing the Sharing Economy

1. **Borrow First**: Before purchasing, check local libraries, friends, or platforms for borrowing options.

2. **Offer What You Own**: Share items you no longer use frequently, such as tools, books, or kitchen gadgets.

3. **Promote Swapping**: Encourage your circle of friends and family to host swaps or join existing events.

4. **Advocate for Sharing**: Educate others about the environmental and financial benefits of collaborative consumption.

Reflective Prompts

1. **What Do You Own?**

   o   List items you rarely use. Could they be shared or swapped?

   o   Identify items you often need but don't own. Could you borrow instead?

2. **Community Connections**:

   o   Who in your neighbourhood or network might benefit from a swap event?

   o   Are there existing sharing platforms or libraries you can join?

3. **Sharing Goals**:

   o   What one step can you take this week to participate in the sharing economy?

Inspirational Quote

"Sharing is the new owning. In a connected world, collaboration is the key to sustainability."

Conclusion

The sharing economy is a simple yet powerful way to reduce waste, save resources, and build stronger communities. By embracing libraries, swap events, and collaborative platforms, you contribute to a culture of mindful consumption and environmental stewardship.

Let's redefine ownership together—because sharing isn't just caring, it's a step toward a brighter, greener future.

Chapter 11

Travel and Zero Waste on the Go

Traveling doesn't have to mean leaving your eco-conscious values behind. With some planning and a shift in mindset, you can explore the world while minimizing waste and supporting sustainable practices. This chapter provides practical tips for eco-friendly packing, choosing sustainable transportation, and making mindful decisions while traveling.

Eco-Friendly Packing Tips: Travel Kits, Reusable Bottles, and Lightweight Essentials

Your journey to zero-waste travel begins before you leave home—packing thoughtfully is key. The goal is to reduce single-use items and opt for reusable, durable alternatives that align with your sustainable lifestyle.

Essentials for an Eco-Friendly Travel Kit

1. **Reusable Water Bottle**

   o   opt for stainless steel or BPA-free bottles.

   o   Stay hydrated and avoid purchasing plastic bottles.

2. **Travel Utensil Set**

   o   Pack lightweight, reusable cutlery made from bamboo or stainless steel.

o   Include a reusable straw and chopsticks for versatility.

3. **Reusable Food Containers**

   o   Bring collapsible silicone or stainless-steel containers for leftovers or snacks.

   o   Perfect for markets, street food, or packed lunches.

4. **Cloth Bags and Produce Bags**

   o   Lightweight and compact, these bags are ideal for shopping or carrying items.

5. **Solid Toiletries**

   o   Choose bar soap, shampoo bars, and conditioner bars to eliminate plastic packaging.

   o   Travel-friendly, TSA-compliant, and long-lasting.

6. **Reusable Makeup Wipes or Cotton Rounds**

   o   Washable alternatives to disposable makeup removers and wipes.

7. **Eco-Friendly Travel Towel**

   o   Lightweight, quick-drying towels made from sustainable materials like bamboo or organic cotton are perfect for travellers.

Tips for Packing Light and Sustainable

- **Pack Versatile Clothing**: Choose layers and neutral colours that can mix and match for multiple outfits.

- **Choose Durable Luggage**: Invest in high-quality bags made from recycled materials or eco-friendly fabrics.

- **Minimize Electronics**: Pack only essential devices and use solar-powered chargers when possible.

By packing with intention, you'll reduce waste, save space, and make your travels more convenient and sustainable.

Sustainable Transportation: Walking, Cycling, and Public Transit

How you get to your destination and move around once there has a significant environmental impact. Opting for sustainable transportation methods can drastically reduce your carbon footprint.

Walking and Cycling

- **Walking**

    o Explore cities and towns on foot to experience local culture and discover hidden gems.

    o Walking is not only eco-friendly but also a great way to stay active during your trip.

- **Cycling**

    o Many cities offer bike-sharing programs for visitors.

    o Cycling is a faster way to navigate while staying eco-conscious.

Public Transit

- Trains, buses, and subways are more energy-efficient and cost-effective than taxis or rental cars.

- Use apps to plan routes and schedules for seamless travel.

- Look for local transit passes for tourists—they save money and encourage you to use public systems.

Long-Distance Travel

1. **Trains and Buses**

    o Choose trains or buses over flights for medium-distance travel.

    o Trains emit significantly less CO2 compared to airplanes.

2. **Carbon Offsetting for Flights**

   o If flying is unavoidable, select airlines that offer carbon offset programs.

   o Pack light to reduce the plane's weight and overall fuel consumption.

Carpooling and Ridesharing

- Use apps like BlaBlaCar or carpool with friends to reduce emissions.

- opt for electric or hybrid vehicles when renting cars.

Sustainable transportation not only lowers your environmental impact but also allows you to immerse yourself in local experiences.

Avoiding Tourist Waste: Choosing Eco-Conscious Accommodations and Dining

Tourism generates an enormous amount of waste, but you can make conscious decisions to avoid contributing to the problem.

Eco-Conscious Accommodations

1. **Green Hotels and Eco-Lodges**

   o Look for certifications like LEED, Green Globe, or Earth Check.

   o Choose accommodations that prioritize renewable energy, water conservation, and waste reduction.

2. **Stay Local**

   o Support small, locally-owned guesthouses, homestays, or Airbnb rentals.

   o This benefits the community and often provides a more authentic experience.

3. **Minimal Room Service**

   o Decline daily housekeeping to save water and energy.

     o   Reuse towels and sheets during your stay.

Sustainable Dining Choices

1. **Eat Local and Seasonal**

   o   Support local farmers and reduce the carbon footprint of imported foods.

   o   Choose restaurants that source ingredients sustainably.

2. **Say No to Single-Use Items**

   o   Bring your reusable utensils, straws, and containers when dining out.

   o   Politely decline plastic straws, cutlery, or Styrofoam containers.

3. **Zero-Waste Dining**

   o   Seek out restaurants that operate with a zero-waste philosophy.

   o   Use apps like "Too Good To Go" to reduce food waste by purchasing unsold meals at discounted prices.

Souvenirs and Shopping

- Choose meaningful, locally-made souvenirs over mass-produced trinkets.

- Avoid items made from endangered species or non-sustainable materials.

- Bring your cloth bag for purchases.

Real-Life Example: Zero-Waste Travel Made Easy

Emma, a frequent traveller and eco-enthusiast, planned a trip to Japan using zero-waste principles. She packed a reusable travel kit, stayed in a solar-powered guesthouse, and explored the cities using a mix of walking and public transit. At restaurants, Emma brought her reusable utensils and avoided disposable chopsticks.

By prioritizing sustainability, Emma not only reduced her environmental impact but also deepened her connection to the local culture and community.

Reflective Prompts

1. **How Can You Start?**

   o   What reusable items can you pack for your next trip?

   o   Which sustainable transportation methods are accessible to you?

2. **Community Impact**

   o   How can your travel choices support local businesses and communities?

   o   Are there eco-conscious accommodations or tours in your destination?

3. **Plan Ahead**

   o   Identify potential waste challenges on your trip and plan solutions in advance.

Inspirational Quote

"Travel is not measured by the miles you cover, but by the footprint you leave behind."

Conclusion

Zero-waste travel is about balancing your desire to explore with your commitment to sustainability. By packing reusable essentials, prioritizing eco-friendly transportation, and making mindful choices in dining and accommodations, you can reduce waste while enjoying richer, more meaningful travel experiences.

The journey to sustainability doesn't end at home—it follows you wherever you go. With every step, you can inspire others to embrace zero-waste travel and create a world where exploration and preservation go hand in hand.

Chapter 12

Building Long-Term Habits for a Zero Waste Life

Embarking on a zero-waste journey is an inspiring and empowering step toward a sustainable future. But to make lasting change, it's essential to turn zero-waste practices into ingrained habits that evolve with your life. This chapter focuses on building a foundation for sustainable living by tracking your progress, adapting to challenges, and inspiring others to join the movement.

Tracking Progress: How to Measure Your Success

To stay motivated, it's important to see the impact of your efforts. Measuring progress not only provides validation but also highlights areas for improvement.

Create a Baseline

Before diving into zero waste, take stock of your current habits:

1. **Conduct a Waste Audit**

   o   Examine your trash for a week. What's in it? What's reusable, recyclable, or compostable?

2. **Set Realistic Goals**

o   Start with achievable targets, such as reducing single-use plastics or composting food scraps.

Use Metrics to Track Progress

1. **Weight of Waste**

    o   Weigh your trash weekly to see reductions over time.

2. **Items Saved**

    o   Track the number of items you've reused or repurposed instead of discarding.

3. **Financial Savings**

    o   Calculate the money saved by using reusable products and minimizing purchases.

Celebrate Milestones

- Reward yourself for hitting goals, such as reducing waste by 50% or completing a month without disposable plastics.

- Share your achievements with family and friends to encourage them to follow suit.

By tracking your progress, you'll gain a clearer picture of how far you've come and where you can go next.

Adapting to New Challenges: Seasonal and Lifestyle Changes

Sustainability isn't static—it requires flexibility to adapt to different circumstances. Life changes, seasons shift, and challenges arise, but your commitment to zero waste can stay consistent.

Navigating Seasonal Shifts

1. **Winter Challenges**

    o   Composting: Keep an indoor compost bin or worm farm during colder months.

o   Energy Efficiency: Insulate your home and layer clothing to reduce heating needs.

2. **Summer Strategies**

o   Stay Hydrated: Carry a reusable water bottle everywhere.

o   Outdoor Events: Bring reusable picnic gear, such as bamboo utensils and cloth napkins.

Adapting to Lifestyle Changes

1. **Moving to a New Location**

o   Research local recycling programs and zero-waste stores in your area.

o   Connect with community groups focused on sustainability.

2. **Family Growth**

o   For parents: Switch to cloth diapers, homemade baby food, and second-hand baby gear.

o   For larger households: Bulk buying and meal prepping can help reduce packaging waste.

3. **Travel and Work**

o   Keep zero-waste essentials in your car or bag for on-the-go needs.

o   Advocate for eco-friendly practices at work, such as recycling bins and digital documents.

Be Kind to Yourself

- Sustainability is a journey, not a race. Give yourself grace when things don't go as planned, and use setbacks as opportunities to learn and improve.

Inspiring Others: Sharing Your Journey and Advocating for Change

Individual action is powerful, but the ripple effect of inspiring others can create a transformative wave of change.

Share Your Story

1. **Social Media**

   o Document your journey with tips, successes, and challenges.

   o Use hashtags like #ZeroWaste and #EcoLiving to connect with like-minded individuals.

2. **Blog or Vlog**

   o Create content that resonates with your community, such as tutorials, DIY guides, or personal anecdotes.

Advocate for Change

1. **Educate Others**

   o Host workshops or presentations on zero-waste practices at schools, workplaces, or community centres.

   o Provide practical tips and starter kits to make it easier for newcomers.

2. **Engage with Local Businesses**

   o Encourage stores to adopt refill stations or reduce packaging.

   o Support businesses that prioritize sustainability.

3. **Collaborate with Policy Makers**

   o Petition for policies that support recycling programs, composting initiatives, or bans on single-use plastics.

Foster a community

- Organize zero-waste challenges or events, such as cleanups or swap meets.

- Create a local zero-waste network where members can share resources, ideas, and support.

By inspiring others, you amplify the impact of your actions and contribute to a collective movement for a healthier planet.

Real-Life Example: Habit Building in Action

Lila, a teacher, began her zero-waste journey by focusing on her classroom. She introduced reusable supplies, created a recycling station, and taught students about sustainability through hands-on projects. The changes inspired her colleagues and students' families to adopt zero-waste practices, spreading the impact far beyond her initial efforts.

Lila's journey shows that even small changes can spark significant transformations when shared with others.

Reflective Prompts

1. **Tracking Your Progress**

   o What's one area of your life where you can measure your zero-waste success?

   o How will you celebrate your achievements?

2. **Adapting to Change**

   o What seasonal or lifestyle changes challenge your zero-waste habits?

   o How can you prepare for these challenges in advance?

3. **Inspiring Your Community**

   o Who in your life could benefit from learning about zero waste?

   o What platforms or events can you use to share your journey?

Inspirational Quote

"The greatest threat to our planet is the belief that someone else will save it." — Robert Swan

Conclusion

Building long-term habits for a zero-waste life is about persistence, adaptability, and community. By tracking your progress, navigating challenges, and sharing your story, you'll create lasting change not only in your own life but also in the world around you.

The journey doesn't end here—every step forward is an opportunity to inspire others and build a future where sustainability is second nature. Let your actions be a beacon for those around you, proving that a zero-waste lifestyle is not only possible but profoundly rewarding.

Conclusion

Your Role in a Zero Waste Future

The journey to a zero-waste lifestyle is not just an individual choice but a collective movement toward a more sustainable and harmonious future. Throughout this book, you've explored the many facets of zero waste—from mindful consumption to sustainable travel, from eco-friendly household solutions to inspiring community initiatives. Now, it's time to reflect on your role in this transformative journey and embrace the power of your actions.

The Ripple Effect: How Small Changes Create Big Impacts

Imagine a single drop of water falling into a still pond. The ripples it creates extend outward, touching every part of the surface. Your zero-waste efforts, no matter how small, have a similar impact on the environment and those around you.

The Domino Effect of Sustainable Choices

1. **Inspiring Others**

   o When you carry a reusable water bottle or bring your own bags to the store, you set an example for others to follow.

o Small conversations about your choices can spark curiosity and action in friends, family, and colleagues.

2. **Reducing Resource Strain**

   o Simple habits like composting or repairing items reduce demand for landfill space and natural resources.

   o Supporting eco-friendly businesses encourages others to adopt sustainable practices.

3. **Cumulative Environmental Benefits**

   o Each time you refuse single-use plastics or conserve energy, you contribute to a larger global effort to reduce pollution and combat climate change.

   o Multiply your actions by thousands of like-minded individuals, and the collective impact becomes monumental.

The ripple effect underscores the truth that even the smallest actions matter. Your choices today shape the world of tomorrow.

Celebrate Your Journey: Recognizing Personal Milestones

Sustainability is a marathon, not a sprint. Recognizing your progress and celebrating milestones keeps you motivated and reminds you of the difference you're making.

Reflect on Your Achievements

1. **What Have You Accomplished?**

   o Look back at the waste you've diverted from landfills, the money you've saved, and the habits you've changed.

2. **How Has Your Perspective Shifted?**

   o Notice how you now see opportunities to reduce waste in everyday scenarios that once felt overwhelming.

Mark Your Milestones

1. **Celebrate Wins Big and Small**

   o   Whether it's a month without single-use plastics or convincing a friend to go zero waste, take pride in your achievements.

2. **Reward Yourself**

   o   Treat yourself to an eco-friendly item you've been eyeing or enjoy a zero-waste picnic with loved ones.

   Share Your Success

1. **Social Media Highlights**

   o   Post about your milestones to inspire others and connect with a community of like-minded individuals.

2. **Encourage Feedback**

   o   Share your challenges and triumphs to foster discussions and exchange tips with others.

Celebrating your journey reinforces the value of your efforts and reminds you of the positive impact you've created.

Call to Action: Commit to a Sustainable Lifestyle

Every great movement begins with a commitment, and living a zero-waste life is no different. Now is the time to take what you've learned and make it a cornerstone of your everyday existence.

Set Your Intentions

1. **Start Small**

   o   Choose one area to focus on, such as reducing food waste or switching to reusable products, and build from there.

2. **Stay Consistent**

   o   Sustainable living isn't about perfection; it's about persistence. Progress over perfection is the goal.

Engage with Your Community

1. **Be a Role Model**

   o   Share your zero-waste practices openly to encourage others to join the movement.

2. **Collaborate**

   o   Organize or participate in local events, such as cleanups, workshops, or swap meets, to amplify your impact.

Advocate for Change

1. **Support Policy Initiatives**

   o   Advocate for bans on single-use plastics or improvements to recycling systems in your area.

2. **Vote with Your Wallet**

   o   Prioritize businesses and products that align with your sustainability values.

Join the Global Movement

1. **Stay Inspired**

   o   Follow sustainability leaders, attend eco-friendly events, and read about environmental advancements to stay motivated.

2. **Pass It On**

   o   Share your journey with future generations, teaching them the importance of preserving the planet.

Your commitment to a zero-waste lifestyle is a powerful statement of hope and action. Together, individual efforts become a collective force for good.

Reflective Prompts

1. **Your Ripple Effect**

   o Who in your life can you inspire to adopt zero-waste practices?

   o What small changes can you implement today to create a larger impact?

2. **Celebrating Success**

   o What milestones have you achieved in your journey toward zero waste?

   o How will you reward yourself for your efforts?

3. **Taking Action**

   o What's one commitment you can make to live more sustainably?

   o How can you engage with your community to spread the zero-waste message?

Inspirational Quote

"Never doubt that a small group of thoughtful, committed citizens can change the world; indeed, it's the only thing that ever has." — Margaret Mead

Conclusion

Your role in a zero-waste future is vital and impactful. By taking small steps, celebrating your journey, and inspiring others, you contribute to a movement that's reshaping the world for the better.

This book has provided the tools, ideas, and encouragement to guide you on your path. Now, it's up to you to take the next step. The choices you make every day—whether it's using a reusable bag, repairing an item, or sharing your story—are acts of care for our planet.

Together, we can create a world where sustainability is second nature and where future generations can thrive. Your journey is just beginning, and the possibilities are endless. Embrace this challenge with hope, determination, and the knowledge that every effort counts.

Let's build a zero-waste future—one thoughtful choice at a time.

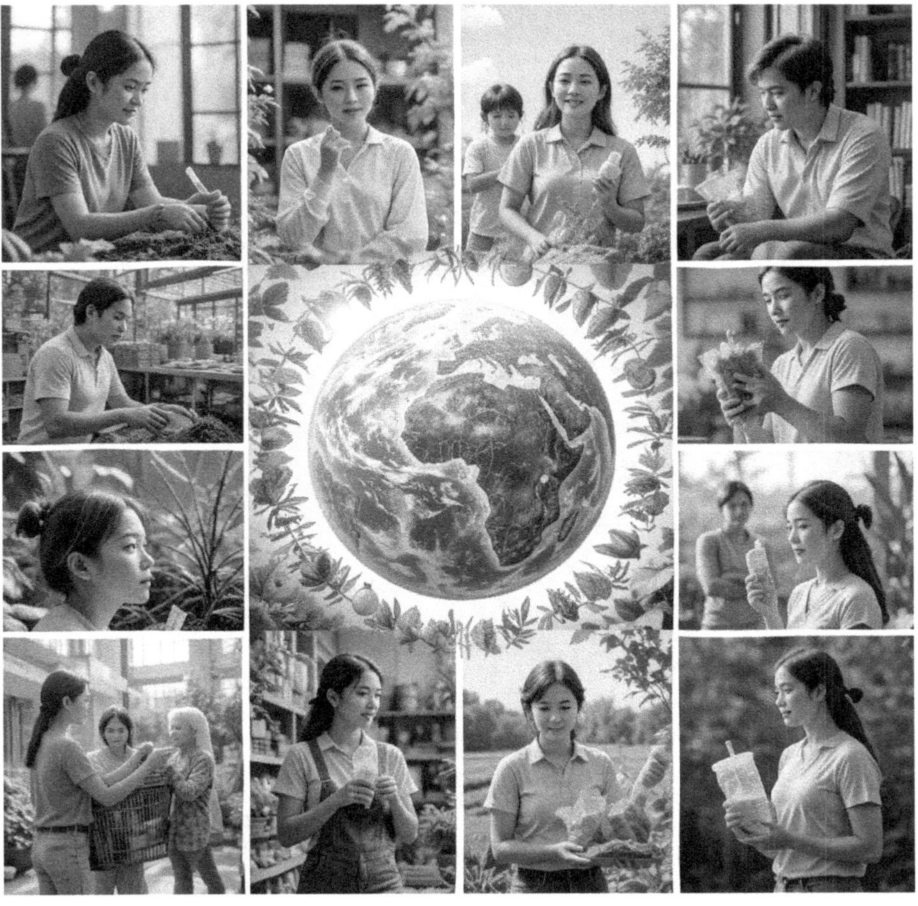